TIMELESS WELLNESS

Navigating Intermittent Fasting for Vibrant Health for Women over Fifty

DR JOYCE A. MOORE

This book does not offer psychiatric or medical advice; it is just intended for informational and educational purposes. If you have specific concerns about your medical or mental health, please speak with a trained expert.

Gratitude

A Grateful Acknowledgment of Your Journey

Thank you for choosing to embark on this transformative journey toward better health and wellness with me. Your commitment to embracing change, caring for your body, and overcoming challenges is truly inspiring. Every step you take today builds a foundation for a healthier, brighter tomorrow.

As you explore the pages ahead, may you discover not only practical guidance and heartfelt encouragement but also the deep strength within you to keep growing and evolving. Each chapter is crafted as a stepping stone on your journey, offering insights and tools to help you navigate challenges and celebrate every small victory along the way. Let the wisdom shared in these pages inspire you to embrace change, cherish progress, and honor the unique path you're on.

Picture a future where every day unfolds with vibrant health and renewed energy—a life where each moment is a testament to your resilience and commitment to self-care. Allow this journey to be a canvas for ongoing self-discovery, where you uncover hidden strengths and develop new ways to nurture your mind, body, and spirit.

Here's to the graceful unfolding of your unique wellness journey—a journey marked by continual learning, mindful practices, and joyful breakthroughs. May each day bring you ever closer to the joy, fulfillment, and lasting well-being you so richly deserve.

With gratitude,

Joyce A. Moore

This Book Belongs To:

Content

Introduction

Welcome to a transforming path of health and well-being designed specifically for lively women over the age of fifty. In this introductory part, we'll look at the basics of intermittent fasting—a powerful approach to nutrition and lifestyle that has the ability to change your relationship with food, renew your energy, and promote long-term heath.

What is Intermittent Fasting?

Intermittent fasting is more than simply a diet; it is a way of life that focuses on when and how much you consume. It entails alternating between periods of eating and fasting, utilizing the body's inherent tendencies to burn stored fat for energy.

As we examine the fundamental ideas, you'll acquire a clear grasp of how intermittent fasting differs from standard diets, providing a sustainable and adaptable strategy to support your health. This eating habit has gained popularity because of its possible health advantages. Unlike other diets, this one focuses on when you eat, not what you eat. It includes alternate fasting and eating periods, comparable to our forefathers' natural feast and famine cycles.

How does it Work?

Unlock the processes underlying intermittent fasting as we explore the complexities of the fasting and eating windows. You'll learn about the science behind intermittent fasting, from hormone changes to metabolic adaptations, and how it may help you lose weight, optimize your energy, and improve your overall health. Learn how this strategy connects with the specific requirements of women over the age of fifty should consider the physiological changes that come with aging.

Contrary to popular belief, it is not about restricting calories or starving oneself when fasting periods are precisely planned, and maintaining a healthy caloric intake during eating windows. Focusing on time rather than limitation fosters a sustainable and healthy relationship with food, resulting in benefits such as weight loss, enhanced metabolic health, and hormonal balance.

Benefits Tailored for Women over Fifty.

Explore the numerous benefits that intermittent fasting especially provides to woman in their senior years. From hormone balancing to weight control to possible cognitive advantages, see how intermittent fasting can provide a bespoke answer for the difficulties and possibilities that may occur at this life period. Let's go deeper into the impact of intermittent fasting, beyond just weight loss. Together, we'll explore how it may influence lifespan, strengthen bones, and enhance mental clarity—factors that truly matter as we age. This isn't about restrictive dieting; it's about discovering a way of eating that feels natural, sustainable, and freeing. Imagine a lifestyle that doesn't just help you manage your weight but also boosts your energy, sharpens your mind, and supports long-term well-being. With the right knowledge and a little commitment, intermittent fasting can become more than just a health trend—it can be an empowering choice that helps you feel your best every day.

So let us go on this journey together. Whether you're looking to improve your health, regain control over your eating habits, or simply feel more vibrant, this approach is designed with you in mind. The benefits of intermittent fasting are not just about food; they're about celebrating and supporting the strength, resilience, and vitality of women over 50. Let's get started!

Chapter 1

The Foundations of Fasting

Begin a thorough and insightful investigation of the basics of fasting where we'll break down the many approaches that fall under the broad umbrella of intermittent fasting. Whether you're new to the concept or looking to refine your current routine, this chapter will serve as your **trusted guide**, helping you navigate the different fasting methods with clarity and confidence.

We'll uncover the unique structures of various intermittent fasting approaches—from time-restricted eating and alternate-day fasting to extended fasts—highlighting their benefits and potential challenges. You'll gain a **clear understanding of how each method works**, what makes them effective, and which approach may best suit your body, lifestyle, and personal goals.

But fasting isn't a one-size-fits-all journey. That's why we'll also explore **key considerations** such as how fasting impacts energy levels, metabolism, and overall well-being—especially for women over fifty. By the end of this chapter, you'll feel empowered with the knowledge to choose a fasting approach that aligns with your needs, supports your health, and feels sustainable in the long run.

Discover the most effective fasting approach for you.

The Different Approaches to Intermittent Fasting

Time-Restricted Eating

Let's take a closer look at **Time-Restricted Eating (TRE)**—one of the simplest and most effective forms of intermittent fasting. This method is easy to follow and works by setting a specific window of time each day for eating while fasting for the remaining hours. By aligning your meals with your body's natural circadian rhythm, **Time-Restricted Eating can help**

regulate metabolism, improve digestion, and support overall well-being. Your body isn't just processing food; it's operating on an internal clock that influences energy levels, hormone production, and even how efficiently you burn calories.

In this section, you'll discover **why meal timing matters** and how following a structured eating window may enhance your health. We can explore different schedules—such as the **16:8, 14:10, or 12:12 methods**—so you can find an approach that fits **your routine, preferences, and goals**.

To make the transition easier, we'll also go over **practical tips** for adjusting your eating window, managing hunger, and ensuring your meals provide the right balance of nutrients to keep you feeling satisfied and energized.

Whether you're looking for a simple way to start intermittent fasting or hoping to fine-tune your current habits, **Time-Restricted Eating offers a flexible and sustainable way to improve your health—without complicated rules or extreme restrictions.**

5:2Method

The **5:2 Method** offers a flexible and manageable approach to intermittent fasting, making it a popular choice for those looking to balance structure with freedom. Unlike daily fasting methods, this approach splits the week into **five days of regular eating** and **two days of reduced calorie intake**—giving you the benefits of fasting without the need for daily restrictions.

The idea behind the 5:2 Method is simple, on five days of the week, you eat as you normally would, focusing on balanced, nutritious meals. On the other two non-consecutive fasting days, you **limit your calorie intake to about 500–600 calories**, allowing your body to shift into a mild fasting state. This cycle gives your metabolism a break while still providing the fuel your body needs.

Throughout this section, you'll learn how the **body responds to fasting days**—from metabolic adjustments to enhanced fat burning and cellular repair. We'll also cover **practical tips for meal planning**, ensuring your fasting days include **nutrient-dense foods** that keep you feeling satisfied and energized.

With its flexibility and ease of implementation, the **5:2 Method** is an approachable way to incorporate intermittent fasting into your lifestyle. Whether you're looking to improve overall health, manage weight, or simply develop a more mindful approach to eating, this method allows you to enjoy the best of both worlds—structure when you need it and freedom when you don't.

Alternate-Day Fasting

This method has gained attention for its potential impact on **weight management, hormonal balance, and metabolic health**. On fasting days, the body shifts into fat-burning mode, improves insulin sensitivity, and may even trigger cellular repair processes. Meanwhile, on eating days, you can enjoy your usual meals, making this approach flexible and adaptable to different lifestyles.

In this section, you'll find **practical strategies** for easing into Alternate-Day Fasting, handling common challenges like hunger and energy dips, and making smart food choices that keep you feeling nourished. We'll cover **how to structure meals** on both fasting and non-fasting days to ensure you're getting the right nutrients while maximizing the benefits of this method.

If you're looking for an intermittent fasting approach that offers both **structure and freedom**, ADF might be the perfect fit—providing a powerful way to support overall health while maintaining a flexible lifestyle.

Modified Fasting

Modified Fasting is a **customizable and adaptable** approach to intermittent fasting that allows you to tailor fasting intervals to fit your personal needs, preferences, and health goals. Unlike rigid fasting methods, this approach gives you the freedom to **adjust fasting durations, calorie intake, and meal timing** based on what works best for your body and lifestyle.

With Modified Fasting, you don't have to follow a strict schedule. Instead, you can explore **different fasting windows**, whether that means **longer fasts on some days and shorter ones on others, partial fasts with minimal calorie intake, or gentle fasting adjustments based on your energy levels and daily demands**. This flexibility makes it easier to incorporate fasting into your routine without feeling restricted.

In this section, we'll explore **how to create a fasting plan that aligns with your lifestyle**, ensuring you still experience the key benefits of intermittent fasting—such as improved metabolism, better digestion, and enhanced overall health. You'll also find **practical tips on meal planning, hydration, and**

nutrient-dense food choices to keep you feeling energized and nourished.

If you're looking for a fasting method that provides structure **without rigid rules**, Modified Fasting offers the best of both worlds—giving you the freedom to make intermittent fasting work for you.

As we navigate through these distinct approaches, envision yourself finding the method that resonates most with your preferences, health objectives, and daily routine. Each approach holds its unique advantages, and in the following chapters, we'll look deeper into the practical aspects of implementing these fasting methodologies, ensuring that your journey is not only effective but also enjoyable. Get ready to embrace the foundations of fasting and discover the path that aligns perfectly with your wellness aspirations.

Extended Fasting

Extended Fasting takes intermittent fasting a step further by **stretching the fasting window beyond the usual daily timeframes**, often lasting **24 hours or more**—sometimes even up to several days. Unlike shorter fasting periods, this approach allows the body to enter **deeper**

metabolic states, unlocking powerful health benefits.

One of the most intriguing effects of Extended Fasting is **autophagy**, the body's natural process of cellular repair and renewal. As fasting progresses beyond a full day, the body switches from using stored glucose to drawing on fat reserves for energy. This can improve metabolic flexibility, aid in fat reduction, and benefit general health.

However, prolonged fasts need careful preparation. In this part, you'll learn about important factors including staying hydrated, maintaining electrolyte balance, and safely reintroducing food after a fast. You'll also learn who may benefit from Extended Fasting, how to proceed with care, and how to heed to your body's cues to guarantee a great experience. Whether you're looking for occasional extended fasts for cellular rejuvenation, intestinal reset, or metabolic advantages, this strategy provides a deeper degree of fasting that, when practiced carefully, may be a powerful tool for long-term wellbeing.

The Warrior Diet - Eating Like Our Ancestors

The **Warrior Diet** is an intermittent fasting approach inspired by the eating patterns of ancient warrior cultures. It follows a **unique structure**—light eating during the day, typically in the form of raw fruits, vegetables, or small amounts of protein, followed by **one large, nutrient-dense meal at night**.

This method is designed to **work with your body's natural circadian rhythm**, allowing for increased alertness and energy during the day while optimizing digestion and recovery in the evening. By **fasting for most of the day**, your body can tap into stored fat for energy, potentially improving **metabolic flexibility, fat loss, and mental clarity**.

In this section, we'll explore the **science behind the Warrior Diet**, including how it affects hormones, digestion, and overall well-being. You'll also learn **practical strategies** for structuring your meals, making sure your evening feast is both satisfying and nutritionally balanced.
For those looking for a **simple yet flexible** approach to intermittent fasting—one that doesn't require strict calorie counting or rigid meal timing—the Warrior Diet offers a practical way to enjoy the benefits of fasting while still feeling nourished and satisfied.

Spontaneous Meal Skipping: An Intuitive Approach to Fasting

Spontaneous Meal Skipping is one of the **most flexible and natural** ways to practice intermittent fasting. Instead of following a strict schedule, this method encourages you to **listen to your body's hunger cues** and skip meals **only when you naturally don't feel hungry**.

Unlike traditional fasting plans that require specific eating and fasting windows, Spontaneous Meal Skipping gives you the freedom to **eat when your body truly needs nourishment and pause when it doesn't**. This can happen for a variety of reasons—perhaps you're not hungry in the morning, too busy to eat lunch, or simply don't feel like having dinner one evening.

This intuitive approach can lead to **several benefits**, including improved **metabolic flexibility, better digestion, and reduced reliance on unnecessary snacking**. However, it's still important to focus on **mindful nutrition** during the meals you do consume, ensuring your body gets the essential vitamins, minerals, and macronutrients it needs.

In this section, we'll explore how to **recognize true hunger versus emotional cravings**, how meal skipping can fit into different lifestyles, and tips for maintaining balanced nutrition without feeling restricted.

For those looking for a **stress-free, adaptable way to incorporate fasting**, Spontaneous Meal Skipping offers an effortless way to reap the benefits of intermittent fasting—without rigid rules or complicated planning.

The Feast-Famine Cycle - Balancing Periods of Eating and Fasting

The **Feast-Famine Cycle** is a **flexible and dynamic** approach to intermittent fasting that mimics natural eating rhythms—**periods of regular eating followed by intentional fasting**. Instead of adhering to a daily fasting window, this method allows you to **vary your eating patterns**, incorporating **days of feasting** (higher calorie intake) and **days of fasting or reduced intake** in a structured way.

This approach provides the body with the **metabolic benefits of fasting**—such as improved insulin sensitivity, cellular repair, and fat burning—while also allowing for periods of **adequate nourishment and recovery**.

Some people follow this cycle weekly (such as alternating feast and fast days), while others adjust it based on their energy levels, workout schedules, or personal goals.

In this section, you'll learn how to **adapt the Feast-Famine Cycle** to suit your lifestyle, whether that means incorporating **higher-calorie days around intense activity or adjusting fasting days for rest and recovery**. We'll also cover **key considerations**, such as ensuring proper nutrition during both feasting and fasting phases, so your body stays fueled and balanced.

As you explore this and other intermittent fasting methods, remember that there is no **one-size-fits-all** approach. **Each method offers a unique way to integrate fasting into your routine**, allowing you to experiment and find what works best for your individual health journey

Chapter 2

Navigating Nutrition during intermittent fasting

Nutrition plays a **crucial role** in making intermittent fasting both effective and sustainable. In this chapter, we'll explore **what to eat, when to eat, and how to optimize your meals** to support your fasting lifestyle. While fasting focuses on **when you eat**, **what you eat** is just as important. The right food choices can **enhance energy levels, support metabolic health, and maximize fasting benefits** like fat burning and cellular repair. From **nutrient-dense whole**

foods to **strategic meal timing**, we'll break down how to fuel your body efficiently.

You'll also discover **how to balance macronutrients**, ensure adequate hydration, and make **smart eating choices** that complement your fasting routine—without feeling deprived. Whether you're fasting for **weight management, longevity, or overall well-being**, this section will provide practical guidance to help you **nourish your body and thrive**.

Balanced Eating for Women over Fifty

As women over fifty navigate the natural changes that come with aging, **nutrition becomes more important than ever**—especially when combined with intermittent fasting. This chapter focuses on the **key nutrients that support bone health, hormonal balance, heart function, and overall well-being** during this stage of life. From **calcium-rich foods** that strengthen bones to **omega-3 fatty acids** that support brain and heart health, we'll explore how to **build a balanced plate** that fuels your body and enhances vitality. You'll learn how to **incorporate protein for muscle maintenance, fiber for digestion, and essential vitamins to promote optimal aging**—all while aligning with your intermittent fasting schedule. This isn't just about eating well; it's about **adopting a nutritional approach that empowers you to feel strong, energized, and vibrant**. By making intentional food choices that work with your body's needs, you can **thrive in this stage of life with confidence and balance**.

Making Nutrition Enjoyable and Sustainable

Intermittent fasting isn't just about when you eat—it's also about **how you nourish your body** during eating periods. This chapter provides **practical tips on meal planning, preparation, and portion control**, ensuring

that every meal is both **delicious and nutrient-dense**.
Imagine a kitchen filled with vibrant ingredients, where **every recipe is a celebration of health and vitality**. With the right approach, intermittent fasting can become an **enjoyable and sustainable lifestyle**, rather than a restrictive challenge.
As we explore this section, you'll discover how to **craft meals that align with fasting principles while honoring your unique needs and preferences**.
Balanced nutrition and intermittent fasting go hand in hand, forming the foundation for **long-term well-being**.
Now, let's dive into some **flavorful**

and nourishing recipes designed to make your fasting journey both satisfying and fulfilling!

Balanced Eating for Women Over Fifty Fasting-Friendly Recipes

Nourishing Recipes for a Balanced Fasting Lifestyle Eating well during your eating windows is just as important as fasting itself. Here are some **delicious, nutrient-dense recipes** designed to fuel your body, support hormonal balance, and keep you feeling energized.

Omega-3-Boosting Salmon Salad

A light yet satisfying meal, packed with **heart-healthy fats, essential omega-3s, and antioxidants**.

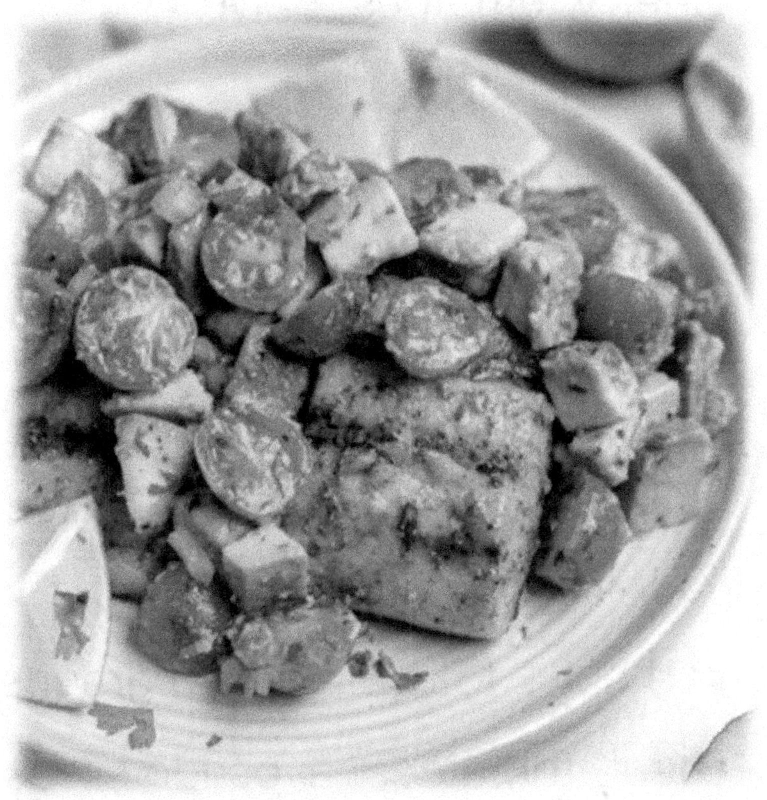

Ingredients:

Grilled salmon fillet

Mixed greens (spinach, arugula, and kale)

Cherry tomatoes, halved

Avocado slices

Walnuts, chopped

Olive oil and lemon dressing

Instructions:

Grill the salmon until cooked to your liking.

In a bowl, toss the mixed greens, cherry tomatoes, avocado slices, and walnuts.

Place the grilled salmon on top.

Drizzle with olive oil and lemon dressing.

 Enjoy a **nutrient-packed meal** that supports hormonal balance and heart health.

Energizing Green Smoothie

A refreshing, antioxidant-rich smoothie is **perfect for breaking your fast** and boosting energy levels.

Ingredients:

Handful of spinach leaves
Handful of kale leaves
½ cup frozen berries (blueberries,

strawberries)
½ banana
1 tablespoon chia seeds
1 cup Greek yogurt or almond milk

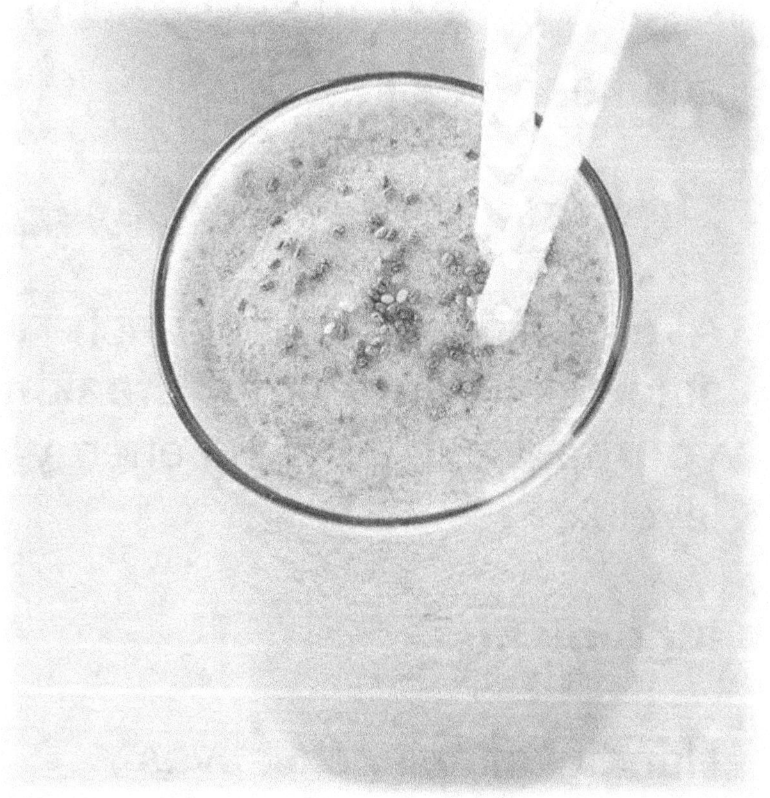

Instructions:

Blend all ingredients until smooth. Pour into a glass and enjoy!

This smoothie is **packed with vitamins, minerals, and fiber**, making it a great way to replenish your body post-fast.

Quinoa and Vegetable Stir-Fry

A hearty and protein-rich meal that provides **sustained energy** during your eating window.

Ingredients:

1 cup cooked quinoa

1 cup mixed vegetables (broccoli, bell peppers, carrots)

½ cup tofu or grilled chicken

1 tablespoon soy sauce

1 teaspoon sesame oil

1 clove garlic, minced

1 teaspoon fresh ginger, minced

Instructions:

Heat sesame oil in a pan and stir-fry the mixed vegetables, tofu, or grilled chicken.

Add cooked quinoa and mix well.

Season with soy sauce, garlic, and ginger.

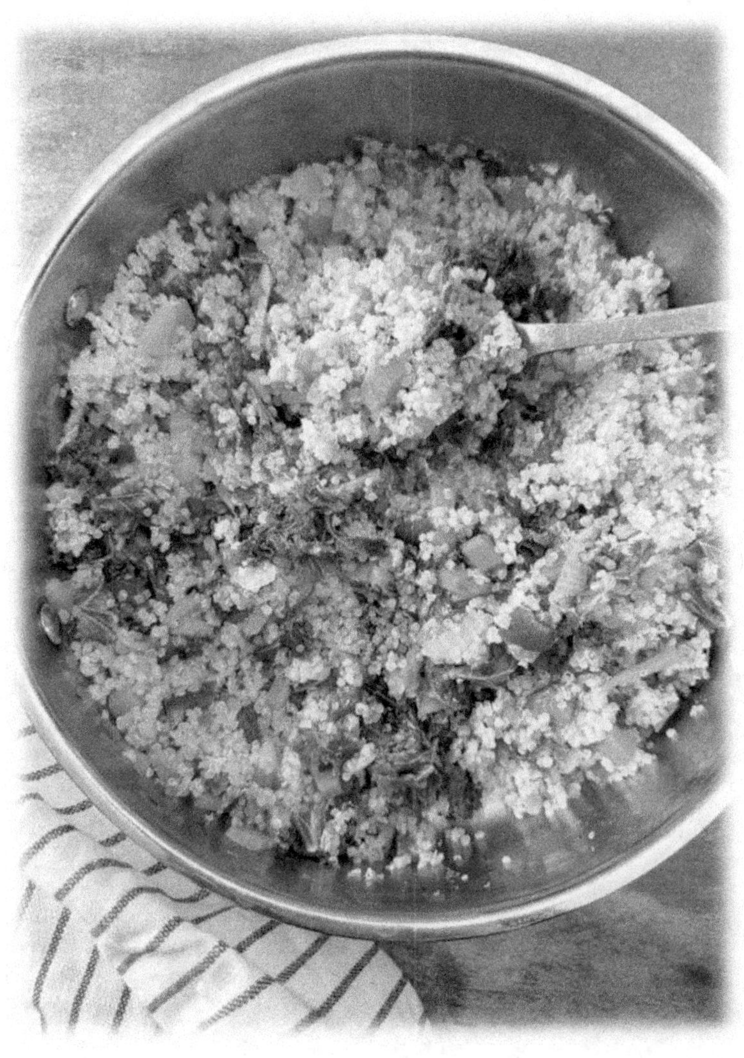

Serve warm and enjoy a **flavorful, nutrient-dense meal**.

These **wholesome recipes** can be adapted to fit your dietary preferences and nutritional needs, offering a **diverse range of delicious options** to support your intermittent fasting journey.

Chapter 3

Optimizing Health through Intermittent Fasting

ntermittent fasting isn't just about when you eat—it's about **how it transforms your entire body and mind**. From balancing hormones and boosting brain function to potentially **supporting longevity and emotional well-being**, fasting goes beyond weight management. This chapter uncovers the **science-backed benefits** of intermittent fasting and how it can help you thrive.

Hormonal Health and Fasting

Did you know that **fasting directly influences your hormones**? It's like a reset button for your body, helping to regulate key hormones that affect **metabolism, energy, and overall well-being**. Here's how:

✔**Insulin Sensitivity:** Fasting helps your body **use insulin more efficiently**, reducing blood sugar spikes and potentially lowering the risk of type 2 diabetes.

✔**Human Growth Hormone (HGH):** Often called the **"youth hormone,"** HGH increases during fasting, helping with **muscle maintenance, fat metabolism, and cell repair**.

✔**Cortisol Balance:** Stress and inflammation can be disruptive, but fasting may help **regulate cortisol levels**, leading to better stress management and hormonal harmony.

For **women over 50**, intermittent fasting may offer **extra benefits** by supporting hormonal shifts during menopause. Many find it helps with **symptom relief, energy levels, and overall well-being** during this life stage.

Intermittent Fasting and Longevity

Can intermittent fasting help you **live longer and age better**? Research suggests that it might! During fasting, your body activates **autophagy**, a natural process where cells **clean out damaged components and regenerate**. Think of it as your body's way of taking out the trash and making room for **healthier, more efficient cells**.

Potential **longevity benefits** of intermittent fasting include:

✔**Cellular repair and renewal** – Helps remove damaged cells and supports overall health.

✔**Reduced risk of age-related diseases** – Research suggests fasting may **support heart health, brain function, and metabolic health**.

✔**Anti-inflammatory effects** – Chronic inflammation is linked to aging and disease; fasting may **help keep inflammation in check**.
By incorporating intermittent fasting into your lifestyle, you're not just **supporting your health today**—you're **investing in a healthier future**.

Intermittent Fasting and Brain Function

Your **brain loves fasting** just as much as your body does! Studies suggest that fasting can **stimulate the production of new brain cells**, leading to:

✔**Improved memory and focus** – Fasting encourages the growth of neurons, helping with **mental clarity and learning**.

✔**Neuro-protection** – Fasting may protect against **age-related cognitive decline**, reducing the risk of conditions like Alzheimer's and dementia.

✔**Brain energy boost** – Ketones (produced during fasting) serve as a **powerful fuel source for brain function**, keeping you sharp and energized.
Think of intermittent fasting as a **brain workout**—helping you stay **mentally agile and alert** as you age.

Emotional Well-being and Intermittent Fasting

Your **relationship with food** is deeply connected to your emotional well-being, and intermittent fasting can play a role in **helping you feel more in control, balanced, and mindful**.

✔**Mindful Eating** – Fasting shifts your focus from mindless snacking to **intentional, nourishing meals**, improving your relationship with food.

✔**Mood Regulation** – Many people report **feeling more stable, less stressed, and more energized** when fasting regularly.

✔**Increased Self-Discipline & Confidence** – Successfully following a fasting routine can lead to **a sense of achievement and self-control**.
When you combine **physical, mental, and emotional well-being**, you unlock a **holistic approach to health**—one where

food, fasting, and lifestyle work in harmony to help you feel your absolute best.

The Bigger Picture

Intermittent fasting is **so much more than skipping meals**—it's a **powerful lifestyle tool** that supports **hormonal balance, longevity, brain health, and emotional well-being**. As you continue this journey, **embrace the flexibility** fasting offers and discover how it fits into your unique lifestyle.

Your **path to vibrant health** is unfolding—one fasting window at a time!

Chapter 4

Overcoming Challenges and Staying Consistent

Intermittent fasting is a powerful tool for health and well-being, but like any lifestyle change, it comes with challenges. With the right strategies, you can navigate these hurdles and make fasting a natural, sustainable part of your daily life. This chapter provides **practical solutions, motivation tips, and strategies for long-term success**, ensuring that fasting becomes not just a habit—but a lifestyle.

Common Concerns and Solutions

When starting intermittent fasting, it's normal to **have doubts, face discomfort, or encounter obstacles**. Here are some common concerns and practical ways to overcome them:

1. Managing Hunger during Fasting Periods

Feeling hungry? Your body is **adjusting to a new eating schedule**. Hunger pangs usually **fade over time** as your body adapts, but in the meantime, try:

✔**Stay hydrated** – Drink **water, herbal tea, or black coffee** to curb hunger.

✔**Keep busy** – Engage in work, hobbies, or exercise to **distract from cravings**.

✔**Eat nutrient-dense meals** – Prioritize **protein, fiber, and healthy fats** in your eating window to stay satisfied longer.

2. Dealing with Social Situations

Fasting can feel tricky when dining with family or attending social events. Here's how to handle it:

✔**Be flexible** – If needed, adjust your fasting window for special occasions.

✔**Communicate openly** – Let friends or family know you're

fasting for health reasons.

✔**Choose wisely** – If eating outside your fasting window, opt for **nutrient-rich choices** that support your goals.

3. Getting Enough Nutrients

Some worry about missing nutrients while fasting. The key is **quality over quantity**—ensure your meals are:

✔**Rich in whole foods** – Include **vegetables, lean proteins, healthy fats, and complex carbs**.

✔**Balanced and filling** – Don't just eat **less**, eat **better**! Prioritize **vitamins, minerals, and**

essential nutrients.

✔**Well-planned** – Prepare meals in advance to avoid **nutrient gaps**.

By addressing these concerns, you'll **gain confidence in your fasting journey** and make it **a smooth, rewarding experience**.

Staying Motivated and Consistent

The secret to long-term success? **Staying consistent**—even on tough days. Here's how to maintain motivation:

✔**Set Realistic Goals** – Define **why** you're fasting (weight loss, energy, longevity) and break it into **small, achievable milestones**.

✔**Track Your Progress** – Use a **journal, app, or calendar** to monitor **fasting hours, energy levels, and results**.

✔**Celebrate wins** – Every successful fast is an **achievement!** Reward yourself with **non-food treats** (new workout gear, self-care, or a fun activity).

Fasting should **fit into your lifestyle**, not disrupt it. The more natural it feels, the easier it will be to **stay on track**.

Nurturing a Positive Relationship with Food

Intermittent fasting isn't about **restriction**—it's about **mindful eating**. Instead of seeing food as something to avoid, fasting helps you **appreciate meals more deeply**.

✔**Listen to Your Body** –
Recognize real hunger vs. emotional cravings.

✔**Savor Your Meals** – Eat slowly, enjoy flavors, and focus on **nourishment, not just calories**.

✔**Break Free from Emotional Eating** – Learn to eat intentionally, **not impulsively**.

Imagine a future where **food brings joy, energy, and balance** rather than stress or guilt. Fasting can help you **redefine your relationship with eating** for the better.

Building a Supportive Community

No one thrives alone! Having a **support system** can make all the difference. Consider:

✔**Joining Online Communities** – Connect with others on social media or fasting forums.

✔**Engaging with Friends & Family** – Share your goals and invite **like-minded individuals** to join you.

✔Finding an Accountability Partner – Having someone to check in with **keeps you motivated**.

Being part of a community **helps you stay inspired, learn new tips, and navigate challenges together**.

Embracing Flexibility and Adaptability

Life is unpredictable, and fasting should be **a tool for health, not a rigid rule**. Learn to **adjust fasting to your needs**:

✔Adapting to Busy Days – If your schedule is hectic, **choose a**

fasting window that fits (like skipping breakfast or eating earlier).

✔**Navigating Special Occasions** – Enjoy celebrations **without guilt** by **shifting your fasting hours** if needed.

✔**Listening to Your Body** – If you're feeling unwell or extra hungry, **adjust as necessary**—consistency matters more than perfection.

A **flexible, adaptable mindset** will ensure intermittent fasting **remains a long-term success** rather than a short-term experiment.

The Road to Long-Term Success

Consistency, balance, and adaptability are **key to making intermittent fasting a lasting lifestyle**. As you continue this journey, remember:

✔**You are in control** – Find a fasting schedule that fits your life.

✔**It is about progress, not perfection** – Some days will be easier than others, and that's okay!

✔**Enjoy the process** – Fasting is about **feeling good, not just following rules**.

Intermittent fasting isn't a **quick fix**—it's a sustainable, empowering approach to **health, energy, and well-being**.

You've got this!

Chapter 5

Beyond Fasting: A Holistic Approach to Wellness

Intermittent fasting is a powerful tool for health, but true well-being extends far beyond when and what you eat. To fully harness its benefits, it's essential to integrate exercise, mindfulness, emotional well-being, and self-care into your lifestyle. This chapter looks into how to develop a comprehensive, balanced strategy that maximizes the transforming impacts of intermittent fasting, leaving you feeling stronger, healthier, and more fulfilled.

Incorporating Exercise into Your Routine

Exercise is more than just a way to stay fit—it **boosts energy, supports mental health, and complements intermittent fasting**. The key is to find movement that **fits your lifestyle, respects your body's needs, and enhances your fasting journey**.

Tailoring Workouts to Support Fasting

Exercising in a fasted state may promote **fat burning, metabolic flexibility, and increased energy levels**. Here's how to structure your workouts:

✔**Light cardio (walking, cycling, or yoga)** – Ideal for fasted workouts, especially in the morning.

✔**Strength training (bodyweight exercises, resistance bands, or weights)** – Helps maintain muscle mass and metabolism.

✔**Flexibility exercises (stretching, Pilates, or mobility work)** – Supports joint health, posture, and balance.

By incorporating **movement that feels good**, you can create **a routine that complements your fasting schedule** and keeps you feeling vibrant.

Mindfulness and Stress Reduction

Your mind and body are deeply connected. Stress can **accelerate aging, impact digestion, and trigger cravings**—all of which can affect intermittent fasting. Cultivating **mindfulness and stress resilience** is key to a sustainable wellness journey.

The Role of Stress in Aging

Chronic stress **increases inflammation and accelerates cellular aging**, making it harder to maintain energy and health. To counteract this:

✔**Prioritize relaxation techniques** – Meditation, journaling, or deep breathing help **lower cortisol levels**.

✔**Get quality sleep** – Poor sleep increases **hunger hormones**, making fasting harder.

✔**Engage in restorative activities** – Reading, spending time in nature, and gentle movement can **calm the nervous system**.

Practices to Enhance Mind-Body Connection

Mindfulness practices help you

stay present, reduce stress, and make fasting feel easier. Try:

✔**Meditation** – Just 5–10 minutes a day can enhance mental clarity and focus.

✔**Deep breathing exercises** – Calms stress and helps regulate hunger cues.

✔**Gratitude journaling** – Shifting focus to positive aspects of life fosters emotional well-being.
A peaceful mind supports a **healthy body**, making intermittent fasting a **joyful experience rather than a challenge.**

Nurturing Emotional Well-Being

Wellness is not just about what you eat—it's also about how you feel about food and your body. Emotional well-being plays a crucial role in making intermittent fasting sustainable.

Embracing Intuitive Eating
Fasting and intuitive eating go hand in hand. Instead of following rigid rules, learn to **listen to your body's hunger and fullness cues**.

✔**Eat when truly hungry** – Not out of boredom, stress, or habit.

✔**Savor every bite** – Enjoy flavors, textures, and nourishment fully.

✔**Let go of guilt** – Food is **fuel and pleasure**, not something to feel bad about.
Intermittent fasting should feel **freeing**, not restrictive. By tuning into your body's natural signals, you **develop a healthier, more intuitive relationship with food**.

Building a Supportive Community

Having **encouragement and accountability** can make all the difference. Find support through:

✔Online fasting groups or wellness communities.

✔Friends and family who share similar health goals.

✔A fasting or wellness mentor for guidance and motivation. Sharing experiences, struggles, and wins **keeps you inspired and connected**.

Embracing Holistic Self-Care
True wellness isn't just about food and exercise—it's about **nourishing your whole being**. A **self-care routine** enhances the benefits of fasting and promotes long-term well-being.

Creating a Personalized Self-Care Routine

Design a self-care plan that aligns with **your needs, lifestyle, and goals**. Consider:

✔**Prioritizing quality sleep** – Aim for 7–9 hours to support metabolism and energy.

✔**Hydration** – Drinking enough water is **crucial for digestion and skin health**.

✔**Skincare and body care rituals** – A simple, nourishing routine promotes **self-love and confidence**.

✔**Journaling and reflection** – Helps track progress, emotions,

81

and insights from your fasting journey.

A **self-care mindset** reminds you that fasting isn't about restriction—it's about **honoring and caring for yourself**.

Exploring Holistic Therapies

Complementary therapies can **support relaxation, digestion, and overall vitality**. Consider incorporating:

✔**Massage therapy** – Relieves tension and enhances circulation.

✔**Acupuncture** – Can balance hormones and support digestion.

✔**Aromatherapy** – Essential oils

like lavender and peppermint promote relaxation and well-being. Experimenting with holistic wellness practices **adds depth and richness** to your health journey.

Adapting to Life's Changes

Life is ever-changing, and a **rigid approach to wellness rarely works long-term**. Instead, embrace **flexibility and adaptability**.
Adapting Fasting to Life Events
Traveling, celebrations, or unexpected life shifts? Instead of stressing, **adjust fasting to fit your life**:

✔**Modify your eating window** for special occasions—consistency over time matters more than perfection.

✔**Practice mindful indulgence**— enjoy treats in moderation, without guilt.

✔**Stay hydrated and focus on nutritious foods**, even if your schedule changes.
Navigating Transitions with Grace
Major life transitions—career shifts, aging, or family changes— can impact well-being. Learn to **adapt without losing sight of your goals**:

✔**Acknowledge changes**

without self-judgment.

✔Focus on what's in your control (sleep, movement, and mindfulness).

✔View challenges as opportunities for growth and resilience.

The key to lasting success is **being kind to yourself while staying committed to your well-being.**

A Lifelong Wellness Journey

True health is a **dynamic, ever-evolving process**, not a destination. When you integrate **fasting, exercise, mindfulness,**

85

emotional well-being, and self-care, you create a **powerful foundation for lifelong wellness**.

✔**Listen to your body and trust the process**.

✔**Be flexible and adapt fasting to your needs**.

✔**Prioritize self-care, movement, and mindfulness daily**.

Intermittent fasting isn't just about changing when you eat—it's about **transforming how you live**. By embracing a **holistic approach**, you unlock **greater vitality, balance, and well-being at every**

stage of life.
You're not just fasting—you're **thriving**.

Exclusive Rejuvenating Juice Collection

As a special bonus with *Timeless Wellness*, enjoy a curated collection of refreshing juice recipes designed to invigorate your body and mind each morning. This exclusive collection offers nutrient-packed blends that help jumpstart your metabolism, deliver vital vitamins and antioxidants, and support hormonal balance—all essential for vibrant health as you navigate intermittent fasting. Each recipe is crafted with the needs of women over fifty in mind, making it easier than ever to enjoy a delicious,

88

revitalizing start to your day. Embrace these juices as a natural boost to your energy, helping you feel refreshed and ready to take on each day with renewed vitality.

1. Radiant Reboot Juice

A green powerhouse to boost energy and support detoxification.

Ingredients:
1 cup kale leaves
1 cup spinach
½ cucumber
2 celery stalks
1 small green apple
½ lemon (peeled)
1-inch piece of ginger

Instructions:
Wash all produce thoroughly.
Chop ingredients into pieces that
fit your juicer.
Process everything through the
juicer.
Stir well and enjoy immediately—
serve over ice if desired.

2. Golden Glow Juice

A vibrant blend rich in beta-
carotene and antioxidants to
brighten your day.

Ingredients:
3 carrots (peeled)
1 orange (peeled)
½ lemon (peeled)
1-inch piece of fresh turmeric (or
½ tsp ground turmeric)

½-inch piece of ginger

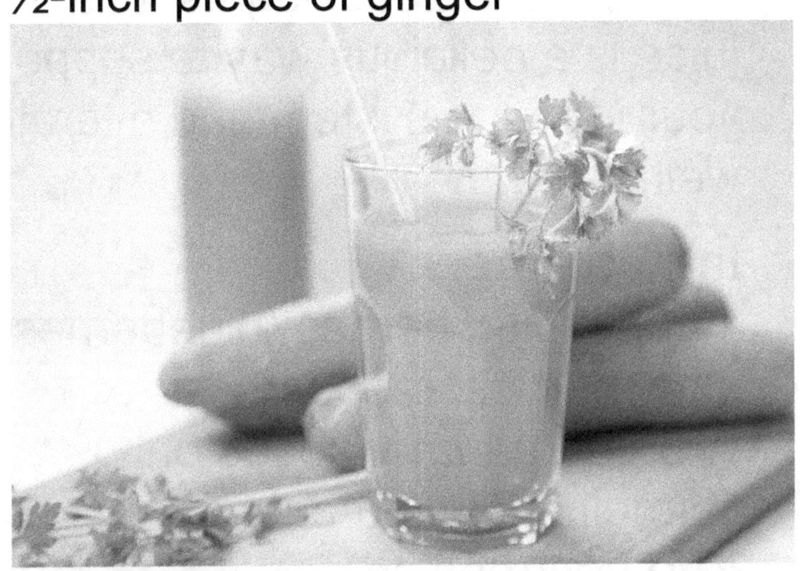

Instructions:

Prepare and peel the carrots, orange, lemon, turmeric, and ginger.
Juice all ingredients together.
Mix well and serve chilled for a burst of golden vitality.

3. Berry Vitality Blend

Packed with antioxidants, this juice is a delicious way to support your immune system and overall well-being.

Ingredients:
1 cup mixed berries (blueberries, strawberries, raspberries)
½ pomegranate (seeds only)
1 small apple (cored)
½ lemon (peeled)
A few fresh mint leaves

Instructions:
Wash all produce and remove the pomegranate seeds.
Combine all ingredients in a blender.

Blend until smooth; strain if you

prefer a smoother texture. Enjoy immediately to get the full benefit of these antioxidant-rich ingredients.

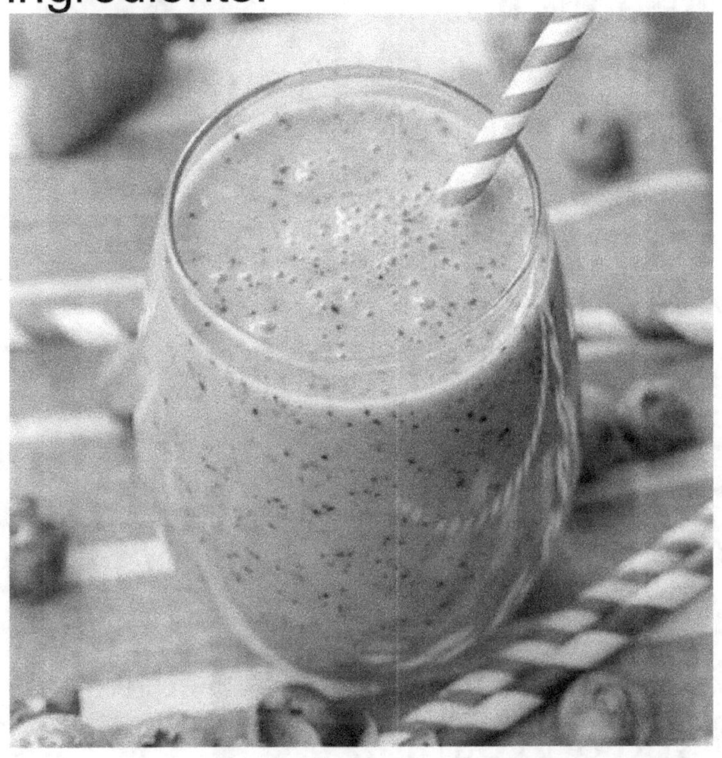

4. Citrus Reviver Juice

93

A refreshing, tangy blend to hydrate, uplift, and kick-start your metabolism.

Ingredients:
1 grapefruit (peeled and segmented)
1 orange (peeled)
½ lemon (peeled)
½ cucumber
A few sprigs of fresh mint

Instructions:
Wash the produce and peel the citrus fruits.
Juice all ingredients together or blend and strain.

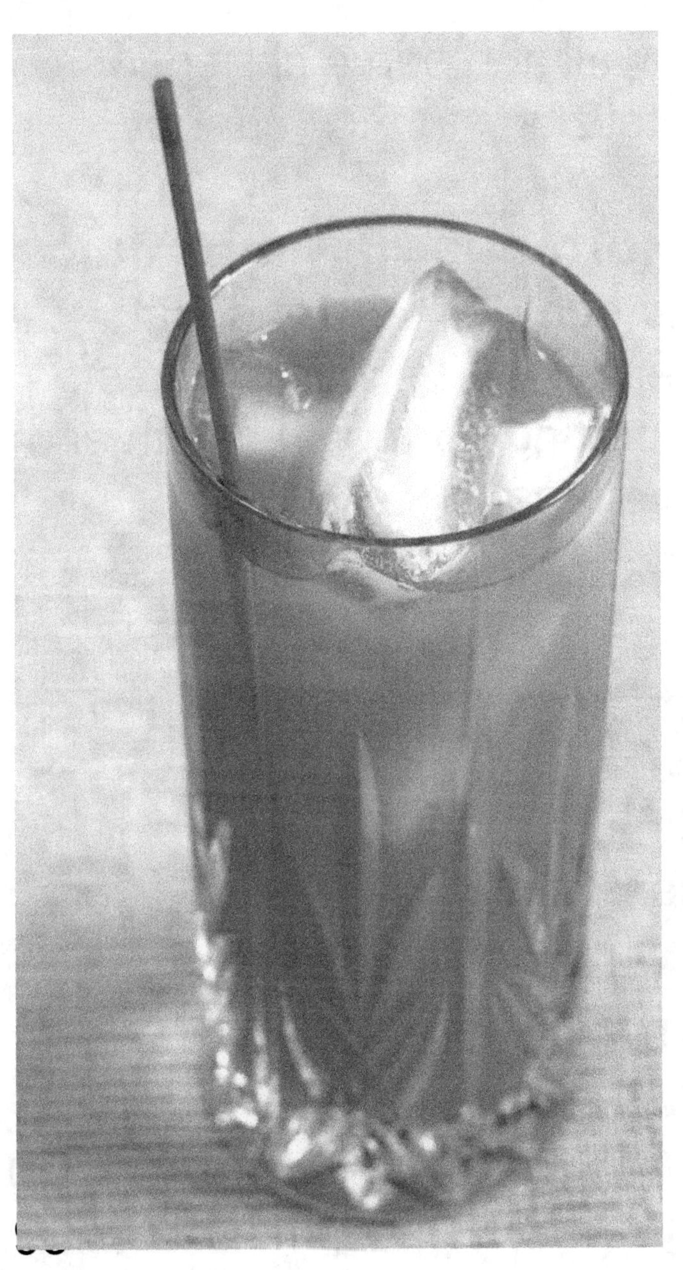

Stir well and serve chilled for a revitalizing start to your day.

5. Hormone Harmony Juice

A nutrient-dense blend that balances earthiness and zest, supporting hormonal health and overall resilience.

Ingredients:
1 medium beet (peeled and chopped)
2 carrots (peeled)
1 small apple (cored)
½ lemon (peeled)
1-inch piece of ginger

Instructions:
Wash and prepare the beet, carrots, apple, lemon, and ginger.

Juice all ingredients and mix thoroughly.
Enjoy the natural sweetness and tang—serve over ice if you like.

6. Watermelon Mint Refresher

A hydrating and delicious juice recipe perfect for a refreshing start to your day.

Ingredients:

3 cups seedless watermelon, cut into cubes
1 small cucumber, peeled and chopped
Juice of 1 lime
A handful of fresh mint leaves (about 8-10 leaves)

Optional: ½-inch piece of fresh ginger (for a subtle kick)
Ice cubes, as needed

Instructions:
Place the watermelon, cucumber, lime juice, mint leaves, and ginger (if using) into a blender.
Blend until smooth.
For a smoother consistency, strain the mixture through a fine mesh sieve into a glass.
Add ice cubes if desired, and stir well.
Enjoy your refreshing and nutrient-packed Watermelon Mint Refresher!
This juice is rich in vitamins, antioxidants, and hydration—

perfect for supporting vitality and well-being.

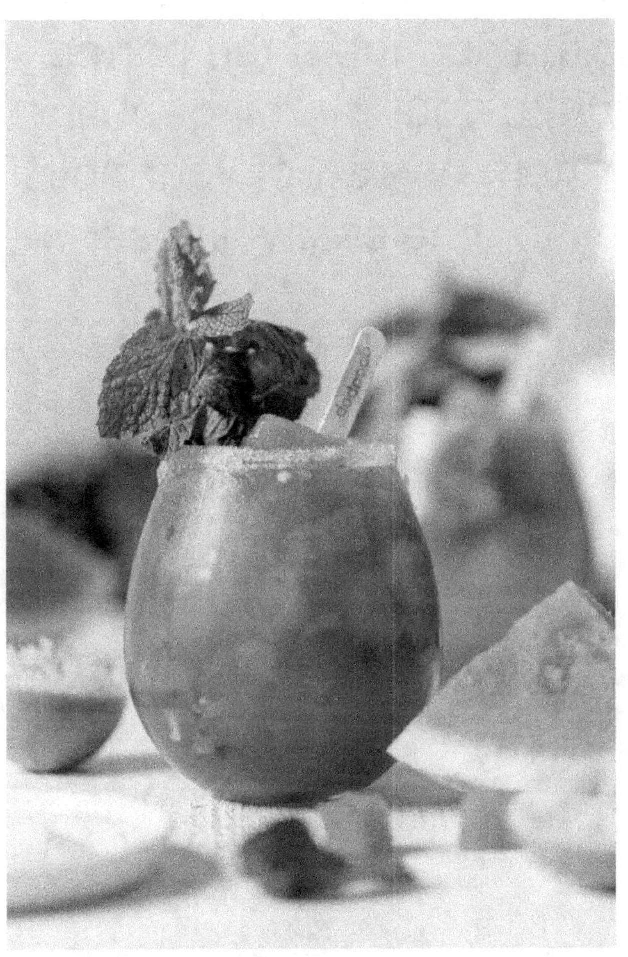

Each of these juices is crafted to provide a burst of nutrients and flavor, making them the perfect addition to your morning routine. Enjoy them as part of your holistic journey to timeless wellness!

Nutrition

& Fasting Journal

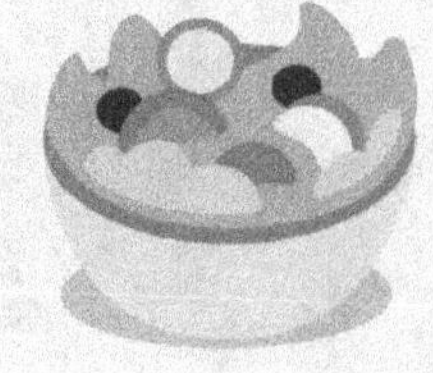

NAME: _________________   DATE: _______________

FASTING DETAILS

FASTING START TIME: ___________________
FASTING END TIME: ___________________
TOTAL HOURS FASTED: ___________________
HOW DID YOU FEEL DURING YOUR FASTING PERIOD?
(ENERGY, MOOD, ANY CHALLENGES, ETC.)

HYDRATION TRACKER

TOTAL WATER INTAKE (CUPS): ___________________
ADDITIONAL BEVERAGES (TEA, HERBAL INFUSIONS, ETC.)

PHYSICAL ACTIVITY

TYPE OF EXERCISE: ___________________________
DURATION: ___________________________
HOW DID IT FEEL?

MEALS & SNACKS LOG

TIME: ___________________
FOODS CONSUMED:
PORTION SIZE/COMMENTS

TIME: ___________________
FOODS CONSUMED:
PORTION SIZE/COMMENTS

Nutrition
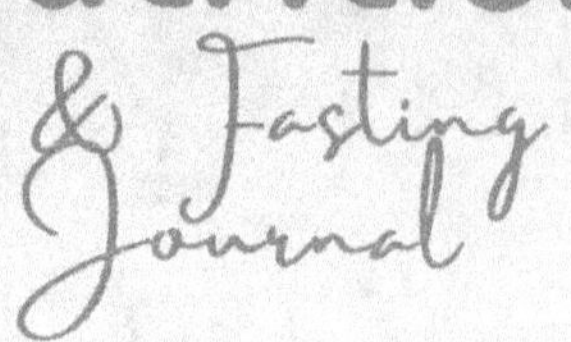
& Fasting Journal

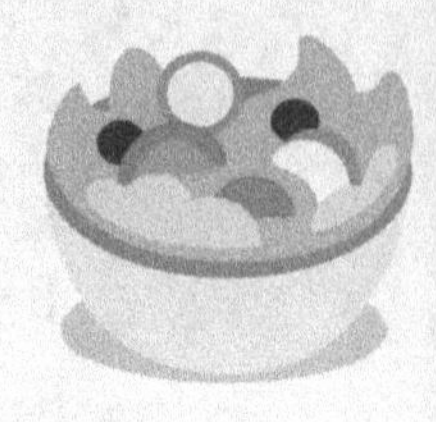

NAME: ________________________   **DATE:** ________________

FASTING DETAILS
FASTING START TIME: _____________________
FASTING END TIME: _____________________
TOTAL HOURS FASTED: _____________________
HOW DID YOU FEEL DURING YOUR FASTING PERIOD?
(ENERGY, MOOD, ANY CHALLENGES, ETC.)

HYDRATION TRACKER
TOTAL WATER INTAKE (CUPS): _____________________
ADDITIONAL BEVERAGES (TEA, HERBAL INFUSIONS, ETC

PHYSICAL ACTIVITY
TYPE OF EXERCISE: _____________________________
DURATION: _____________________________
HOW DID IT FEEL?

MEALS & SNACKS LOG

TIME: _____________________
FOODS CONSUMED:
PORTION SIZE/COMMENTS

TIME: _____________________
FOODS CONSUMED:
PORTION SIZE/COMMENTS

Nutrition

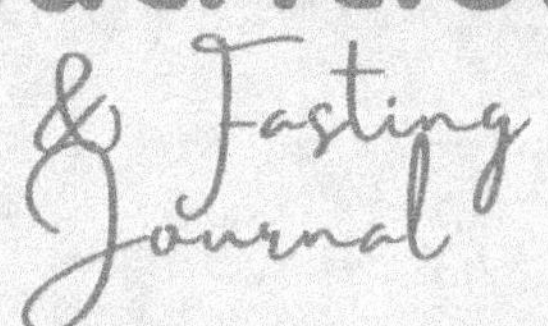

& Fasting Journal

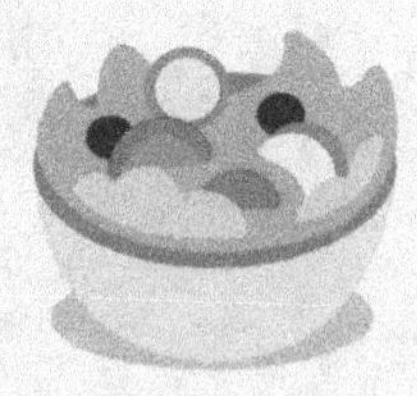

NAME: _______________________   **DATE:** _______________

FASTING DETAILS
FASTING START TIME: _______________________
FASTING END TIME: _______________________
TOTAL HOURS FASTED: _______________________
HOW DID YOU FEEL DURING YOUR FASTING PERIOD?
(ENERGY, MOOD, ANY CHALLENGES, ETC.)

HYDRATION TRACKER
TOTAL WATER INTAKE (CUPS): _______________________
ADDITIONAL BEVERAGES (TEA, HERBAL INFUSIONS, ETC.)

PHYSICAL ACTIVITY
TYPE OF EXERCISE: _______________________
DURATION: _______________________
HOW DID IT FEEL?

MEALS & SNACKS LOG

TIME: _______________________
FOODS CONSUMED:
PORTION SIZE/COMMENTS

TIME: _______________________
FOODS CONSUMED:
PORTION SIZE/COMMENTS

Nutrition
& Fasting Journal

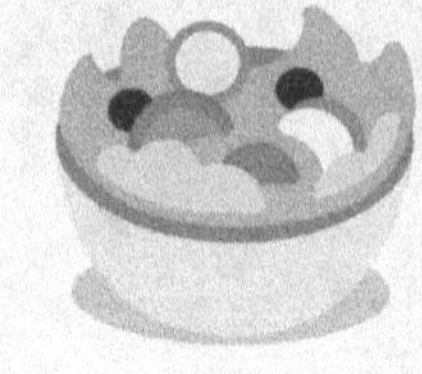

NAME: _________________   **DATE:** _________________

FASTING DETAILS
FASTING START TIME: _________________
FASTING END TIME: _________________
TOTAL HOURS FASTED: _________________
HOW DID YOU FEEL DURING YOUR FASTING PERIOD?
(ENERGY, MOOD, ANY CHALLENGES, ETC.)

HYDRATION TRACKER
TOTAL WATER INTAKE (CUPS): _________________
ADDITIONAL BEVERAGES (TEA, HERBAL INFUSIONS, ETC.

PHYSICAL ACTIVITY
TYPE OF EXERCISE: _________________________
DURATION: _____________________________
HOW DID IT FEEL?

MEALS & SNACKS LOG
TIME: _________________
FOODS CONSUMED:
PORTION SIZE/COMMENTS

TIME: _________________
FOODS CONSUMED:
PORTION SIZE/COMMENTS

Nutrition

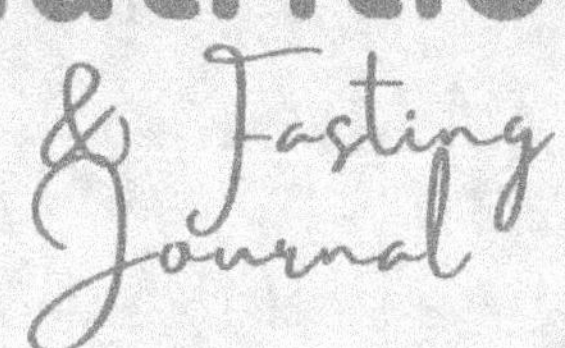

& Fasting Journal

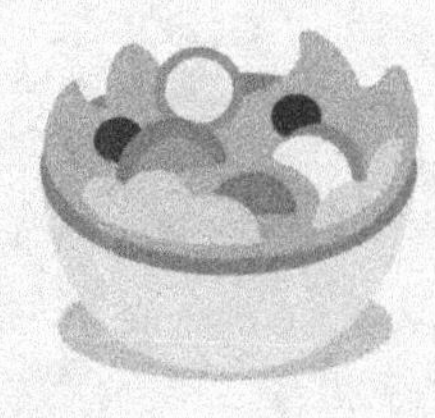

NAME: _________________ DATE: _____________

FASTING DETAILS
FASTING START TIME: _____________________
FASTING END TIME: _____________________
TOTAL HOURS FASTED: _____________________
HOW DID YOU FEEL DURING YOUR FASTING PERIOD?
(ENERGY, MOOD, ANY CHALLENGES, ETC.)

HYDRATION TRACKER
TOTAL WATER INTAKE (CUPS): _____________________
ADDITIONAL BEVERAGES (TEA, HERBAL INFUSIONS, ETC.)

PHYSICAL ACTIVITY
TYPE OF EXERCISE: _______________________________
DURATION: _______________________________
HOW DID IT FEEL?

MEALS & SNACKS LOG
TIME: _____________________
FOODS CONSUMED:
PORTION SIZE/COMMENTS

TIME: _____________________
FOODS CONSUMED:
PORTION SIZE/COMMENTS

Nutrition

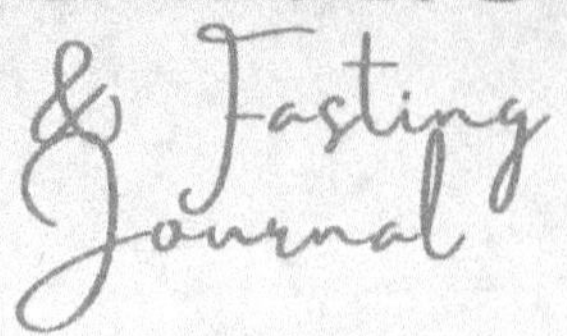

& Fasting Journal

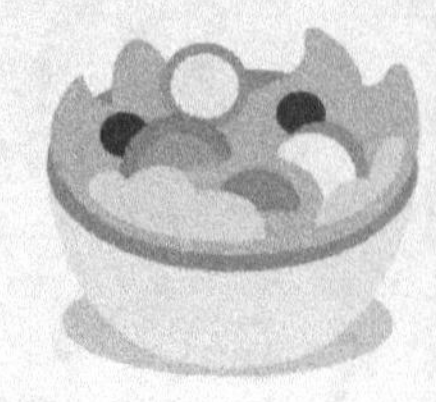

NAME: _________________________   DATE: _________________

FASTING DETAILS

FASTING START TIME: _____________________

FASTING END TIME: _____________________

TOTAL HOURS FASTED: _____________________

HOW DID YOU FEEL DURING YOUR FASTING PERIOD?
(ENERGY, MOOD, ANY CHALLENGES, ETC.)

HYDRATION TRACKER

TOTAL WATER INTAKE (CUPS): _____________________

ADDITIONAL BEVERAGES (TEA, HERBAL INFUSIONS, ETC

PHYSICAL ACTIVITY

TYPE OF EXERCISE: _____________________________

DURATION: _____________________________

HOW DID IT FEEL?

MEALS & SNACKS LOG

TIME: _____________________

FOODS CONSUMED:

PORTION SIZE/COMMENTS

TIME: _____________________

FOODS CONSUMED:

PORTION SIZE/COMMENTS

Nutrition
& Fasting Journal

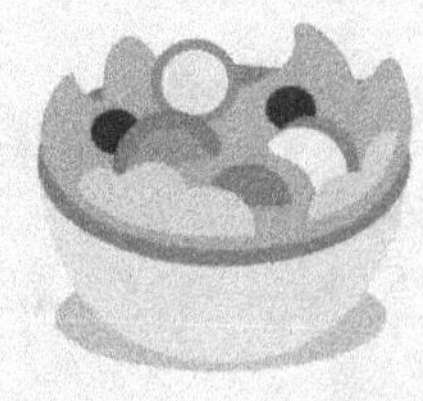

NAME: _______________   **DATE:** _____________

FASTING DETAILS
FASTING START TIME: _____________________
FASTING END TIME: _____________________
TOTAL HOURS FASTED: _____________________
HOW DID YOU FEEL DURING YOUR FASTING PERIOD?
(ENERGY, MOOD, ANY CHALLENGES, ETC.)

HYDRATION TRACKER
TOTAL WATER INTAKE (CUPS): _____________________
ADDITIONAL BEVERAGES (TEA, HERBAL INFUSIONS, ETC.)

PHYSICAL ACTIVITY
TYPE OF EXERCISE: _________________________________
DURATION: _____________________________________
HOW DID IT FEEL?

MEALS & SNACKS LOG

TIME: _____________________
FOODS CONSUMED:
PORTION SIZE/COMMENTS

TIME: _____________________
FOODS CONSUMED:
PORTION SIZE/COMMENTS

Nutrition
& Fasting
Journal

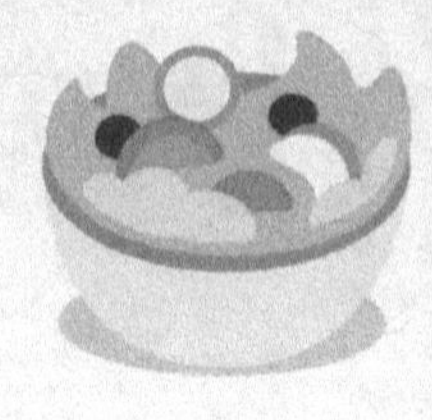

NAME: ________________________   DATE: ________________

FASTING DETAILS
FASTING START TIME: __________________
FASTING END TIME: __________________
TOTAL HOURS FASTED: __________________
HOW DID YOU FEEL DURING YOUR FASTING PERIOD?
(ENERGY, MOOD, ANY CHALLENGES, ETC.)

HYDRATION TRACKER
TOTAL WATER INTAKE (CUPS): __________________
ADDITIONAL BEVERAGES (TEA, HERBAL INFUSIONS, ETC

PHYSICAL ACTIVITY
TYPE OF EXERCISE: ______________________________
DURATION: ______________________________
HOW DID IT FEEL?

MEALS & SNACKS LOG

TIME: __________________
FOODS CONSUMED:
PORTION SIZE/COMMENTS

TIME: __________________
FOODS CONSUMED:
PORTION SIZE/COMMENTS

Nutrition
& Fasting Journal

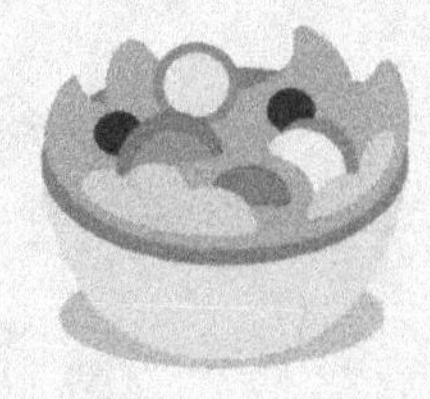

NAME: ___________________   **DATE:** _______________

FASTING DETAILS

FASTING START TIME: ____________________

FASTING END TIME: ____________________

TOTAL HOURS FASTED: ____________________

HOW DID YOU FEEL DURING YOUR FASTING PERIOD?
(ENERGY, MOOD, ANY CHALLENGES, ETC.)

HYDRATION TRACKER

TOTAL WATER INTAKE (CUPS): ____________________

ADDITIONAL BEVERAGES (TEA, HERBAL INFUSIONS, ETC.)

PHYSICAL ACTIVITY

TYPE OF EXERCISE: ____________________________________

DURATION: ____________________________________

HOW DID IT FEEL?

MEALS & SNACKS LOG

TIME: ____________________

FOODS CONSUMED:

PORTION SIZE/COMMENTS

TIME: ________________

FOODS CONSUMED:

PORTION SIZE/COMMENTS

Nutrition
& Fasting Journal

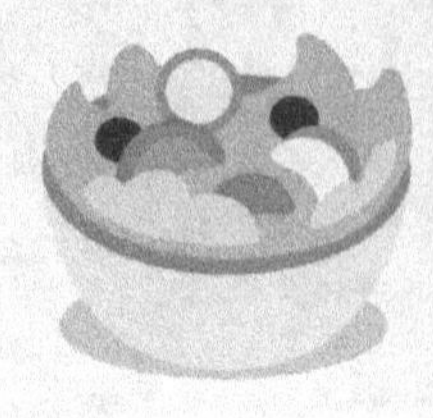

NAME: _______________   **DATE:** _______________

FASTING DETAILS
FASTING START TIME: _______________________
FASTING END TIME: _______________________
TOTAL HOURS FASTED: _______________________
HOW DID YOU FEEL DURING YOUR FASTING PERIOD?
(ENERGY, MOOD, ANY CHALLENGES, ETC.)

HYDRATION TRACKER
TOTAL WATER INTAKE (CUPS): _______________________
ADDITIONAL BEVERAGES (TEA, HERBAL INFUSIONS, ETC

PHYSICAL ACTIVITY
TYPE OF EXERCISE: _______________________________
DURATION: _______________________________
HOW DID IT FEEL?

MEALS & SNACKS LOG

TIME: _______________________
FOODS CONSUMED:
PORTION SIZE/COMMENTS

TIME: _______________________
FOODS CONSUMED:
PORTION SIZE/COMMENTS

Nutrition

& Fasting Journal

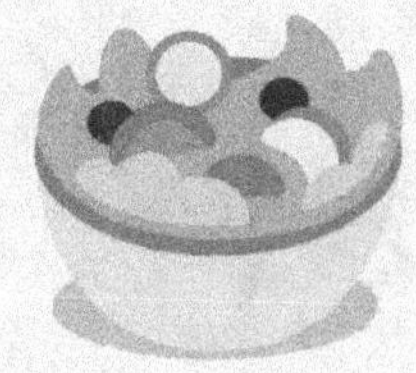

NAME: _________________   DATE: _______________

FASTING DETAILS

FASTING START TIME: _____________________

FASTING END TIME: _____________________

TOTAL HOURS FASTED: _____________________

HOW DID YOU FEEL DURING YOUR FASTING PERIOD?
(ENERGY, MOOD, ANY CHALLENGES, ETC.)

HYDRATION TRACKER

TOTAL WATER INTAKE (CUPS): _____________________

ADDITIONAL BEVERAGES (TEA, HERBAL INFUSIONS, ETC.)

PHYSICAL ACTIVITY

TYPE OF EXERCISE: _______________________________

DURATION: _______________________________

HOW DID IT FEEL?

MEALS & SNACKS LOG

TIME: _____________________

FOODS CONSUMED:

PORTION SIZE/COMMENTS

TIME: _____________________

FOODS CONSUMED:

PORTION SIZE/COMMENTS

Nutrition & Fasting Journal

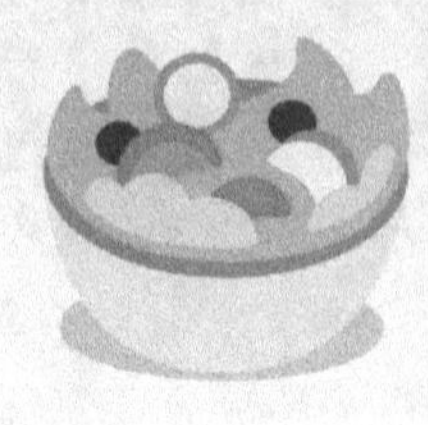

NAME: _________________   **DATE:** _____________

FASTING DETAILS
FASTING START TIME: _____________________
FASTING END TIME: _____________________
TOTAL HOURS FASTED: _____________________
HOW DID YOU FEEL DURING YOUR FASTING PERIOD?
(ENERGY, MOOD, ANY CHALLENGES, ETC.)

HYDRATION TRACKER
TOTAL WATER INTAKE (CUPS): _____________________
ADDITIONAL BEVERAGES (TEA, HERBAL INFUSIONS, ETC.

PHYSICAL ACTIVITY
TYPE OF EXERCISE: _______________________________
DURATION: _______________________________
HOW DID IT FEEL?

MEALS & SNACKS LOG

TIME: _____________________
FOODS CONSUMED:
PORTION SIZE/COMMENTS

TIME: _____________________
FOODS CONSUMED:
PORTION SIZE/COMMENTS

Nutrition

& Fasting Journal

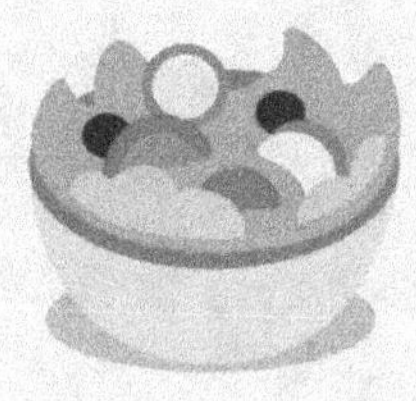

NAME: _________________________   DATE: _________________

FASTING DETAILS

FASTING START TIME: ___________________.

FASTING END TIME: ___________________

TOTAL HOURS FASTED: ___________________

HOW DID YOU FEEL DURING YOUR FASTING PERIOD?
(ENERGY, MOOD, ANY CHALLENGES, ETC.)

HYDRATION TRACKER

TOTAL WATER INTAKE (CUPS): ___________________

ADDITIONAL BEVERAGES (TEA, HERBAL INFUSIONS, ETC.)

PHYSICAL ACTIVITY

TYPE OF EXERCISE: ________________________________

DURATION: ________________________________

HOW DID IT FEEL?

MEALS & SNACKS LOG

TIME: ___________________

FOODS CONSUMED:

PORTION SIZE/COMMENTS

TIME: ___________________

FOODS CONSUMED:

PORTION SIZE/COMMENTS

Nutrition

& Fasting Journal

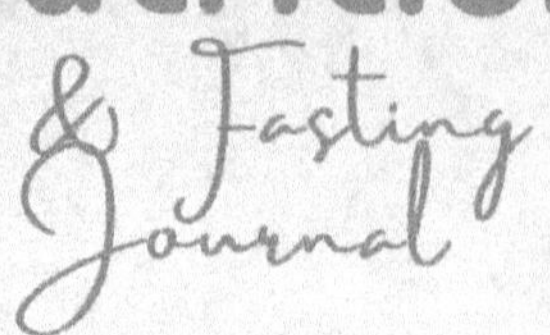
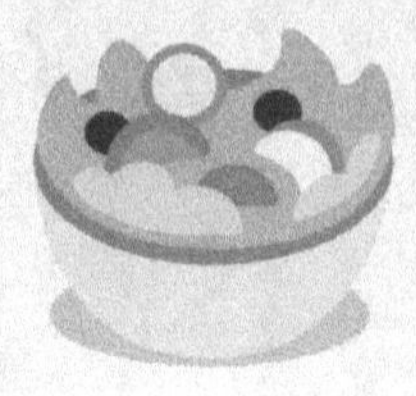

NAME: ___________________   DATE: ___________________

FASTING DETAILS

FASTING START TIME: ___________________
FASTING END TIME: ___________________
TOTAL HOURS FASTED: ___________________
HOW DID YOU FEEL DURING YOUR FASTING PERIOD?
(ENERGY, MOOD, ANY CHALLENGES, ETC.)

HYDRATION TRACKER

TOTAL WATER INTAKE (CUPS): ___________________
ADDITIONAL BEVERAGES (TEA, HERBAL INFUSIONS, ETC.

PHYSICAL ACTIVITY

TYPE OF EXERCISE: ___________________
DURATION: ___________________
HOW DID IT FEEL?

MEALS & SNACKS LOG

TIME: ___________________
FOODS CONSUMED:
PORTION SIZE/COMMENTS

TIME: ___________________
FOODS CONSUMED:
PORTION SIZE/COMMENTS

Nutrition & Fasting Journal

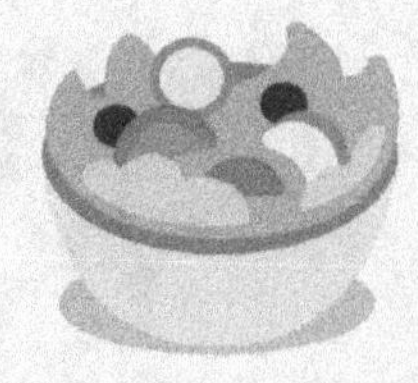

NAME: _________________________   DATE: _______________

FASTING DETAILS

FASTING START TIME: ___________________

FASTING END TIME: ___________________

TOTAL HOURS FASTED: ___________________

HOW DID YOU FEEL DURING YOUR FASTING PERIOD?
(ENERGY, MOOD, ANY CHALLENGES, ETC.)

HYDRATION TRACKER

TOTAL WATER INTAKE (CUPS): ___________________

ADDITIONAL BEVERAGES (TEA, HERBAL INFUSIONS, ETC.)

PHYSICAL ACTIVITY

TYPE OF EXERCISE: _______________________________

DURATION: ___________________________

HOW DID IT FEEL?

MEALS & SNACKS LOG

TIME: ___________________

FOODS CONSUMED:

PORTION SIZE/COMMENTS

TIME: ___________________

FOODS CONSUMED:

PORTION SIZE/COMMENTS

Nutrition

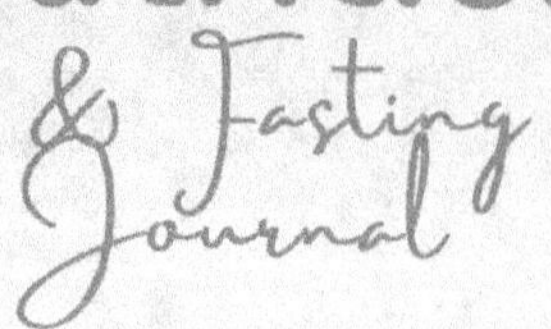

& Fasting Journal

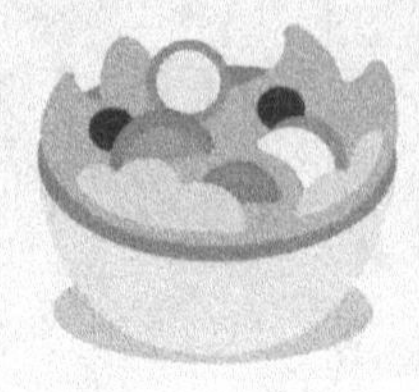

NAME: _______________   DATE: _______________

FASTING DETAILS

FASTING START TIME: _________________

FASTING END TIME: _________________

TOTAL HOURS FASTED: _________________

HOW DID YOU FEEL DURING YOUR FASTING PERIOD?
(ENERGY, MOOD, ANY CHALLENGES, ETC.)

HYDRATION TRACKER

TOTAL WATER INTAKE (CUPS): _________________

ADDITIONAL BEVERAGES (TEA, HERBAL INFUSIONS, ETC.

PHYSICAL ACTIVITY

TYPE OF EXERCISE: _____________________________

DURATION: _____________________________

HOW DID IT FEEL?

MEALS & SNACKS LOG

TIME: _________________

FOODS CONSUMED:

PORTION SIZE/COMMENTS

TIME: _________________

FOODS CONSUMED:

PORTION SIZE/COMMENTS

Nutrition
& Fasting Journal

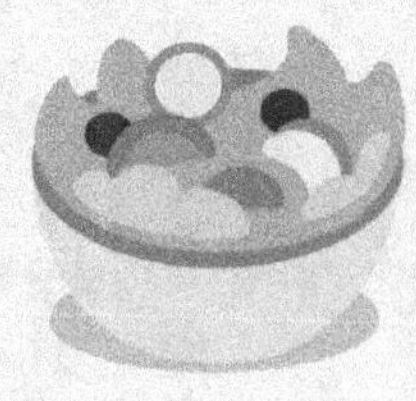

NAME: _________________   **DATE:** _______________

FASTING DETAILS
FASTING START TIME: _________________________
FASTING END TIME: _________________________
TOTAL HOURS FASTED: _________________________
HOW DID YOU FEEL DURING YOUR FASTING PERIOD?
(ENERGY, MOOD, ANY CHALLENGES, ETC.)

HYDRATION TRACKER
TOTAL WATER INTAKE (CUPS): _________________________
ADDITIONAL BEVERAGES (TEA, HERBAL INFUSIONS, ETC.)

PHYSICAL ACTIVITY
TYPE OF EXERCISE: _________________________________
DURATION: _________________________________
HOW DID IT FEEL?

MEALS & SNACKS LOG

TIME: _________________________
FOODS CONSUMED:
PORTION SIZE/COMMENTS

TIME: _________________________
FOODS CONSUMED:
PORTION SIZE/COMMENTS

Nutrition
& Fasting Journal

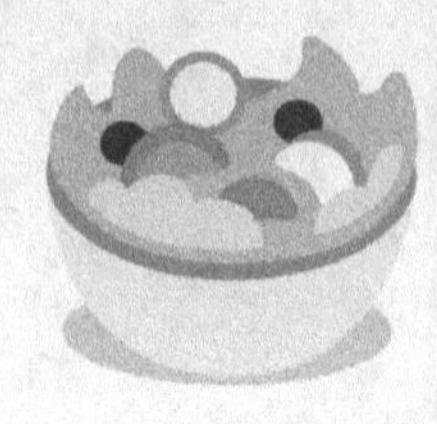

NAME: _________________   DATE: _________________

FASTING DETAILS
FASTING START TIME: _________________
FASTING END TIME: _________________
TOTAL HOURS FASTED: _________________
HOW DID YOU FEEL DURING YOUR FASTING PERIOD?
(ENERGY, MOOD, ANY CHALLENGES, ETC.)

HYDRATION TRACKER
TOTAL WATER INTAKE (CUPS): _________________
ADDITIONAL BEVERAGES (TEA, HERBAL INFUSIONS, ETC

PHYSICAL ACTIVITY
TYPE OF EXERCISE: _________________________
DURATION: _____________________________
HOW DID IT FEEL?

MEALS & SNACKS LOG
TIME: _________________
FOODS CONSUMED:
PORTION SIZE/COMMENTS

TIME: _________________
FOODS CONSUMED:
PORTION SIZE/COMMENTS

Nutrition & Fasting Journal

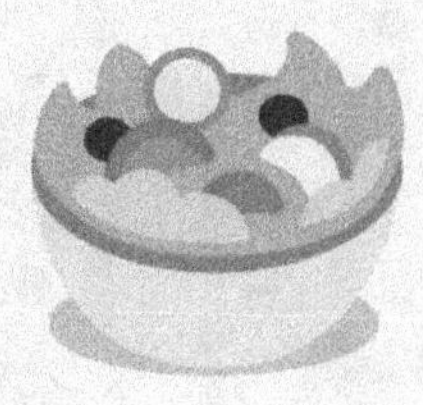

NAME: ________________   DATE: ____________

FASTING DETAILS

FASTING START TIME: ____________________

FASTING END TIME: ____________________

TOTAL HOURS FASTED: ____________________

HOW DID YOU FEEL DURING YOUR FASTING PERIOD?
(ENERGY, MOOD, ANY CHALLENGES, ETC.)

HYDRATION TRACKER

TOTAL WATER INTAKE (CUPS): ____________________

ADDITIONAL BEVERAGES (TEA, HERBAL INFUSIONS, ETC.)

PHYSICAL ACTIVITY

TYPE OF EXERCISE: ____________________________________

DURATION: ____________________________________

HOW DID IT FEEL?

MEALS & SNACKS LOG

TIME: ____________________

FOODS CONSUMED:

PORTION SIZE/COMMENTS

TIME: ____________________

FOODS CONSUMED:

PORTION SIZE/COMMENTS

Nutrition

& Fasting Journal

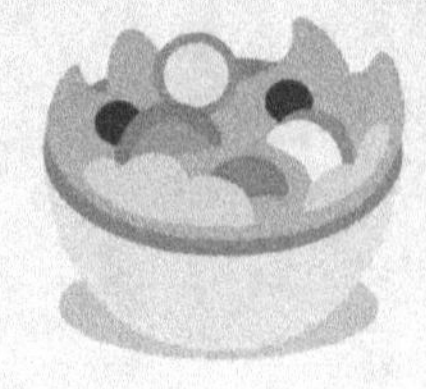

NAME: ___________________   **DATE:** ___________________

FASTING DETAILS

FASTING START TIME: ___________________
FASTING END TIME: ___________________
TOTAL HOURS FASTED: ___________________
HOW DID YOU FEEL DURING YOUR FASTING PERIOD?
(ENERGY, MOOD, ANY CHALLENGES, ETC.)

HYDRATION TRACKER

TOTAL WATER INTAKE (CUPS): ___________________
ADDITIONAL BEVERAGES (TEA, HERBAL INFUSIONS, ETC.

PHYSICAL ACTIVITY

TYPE OF EXERCISE: ___________________
DURATION: ___________________
HOW DID IT FEEL?

MEALS & SNACKS LOG

TIME: ___________________
FOODS CONSUMED:
PORTION SIZE/COMMENTS

TIME: ___________________
FOODS CONSUMED:
PORTION SIZE/COMMENTS

Nutrition

& Fasting Journal

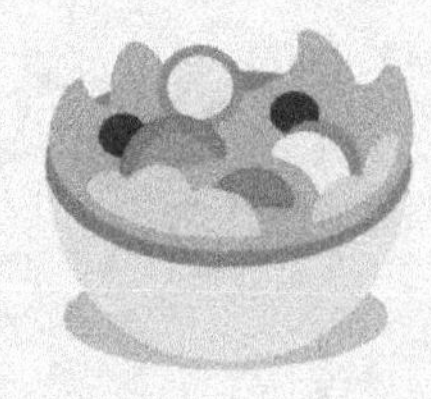

NAME: _______________________   **DATE:** _______________

FASTING DETAILS
FASTING START TIME: _______________________
FASTING END TIME: _______________________
TOTAL HOURS FASTED: _______________________
HOW DID YOU FEEL DURING YOUR FASTING PERIOD?
(ENERGY, MOOD, ANY CHALLENGES, ETC.)

HYDRATION TRACKER
TOTAL WATER INTAKE (CUPS): _______________________
ADDITIONAL BEVERAGES (TEA, HERBAL INFUSIONS, ETC.)

PHYSICAL ACTIVITY
TYPE OF EXERCISE: _______________________
DURATION: _______________________
HOW DID IT FEEL?

MEALS & SNACKS LOG

TIME: _______________________
FOODS CONSUMED:
PORTION SIZE/COMMENTS

TIME: _______________________
FOODS CONSUMED:
PORTION SIZE/COMMENTS

Nutrition

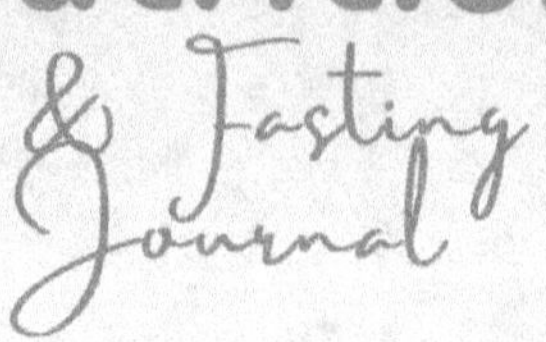

& Fasting Journal

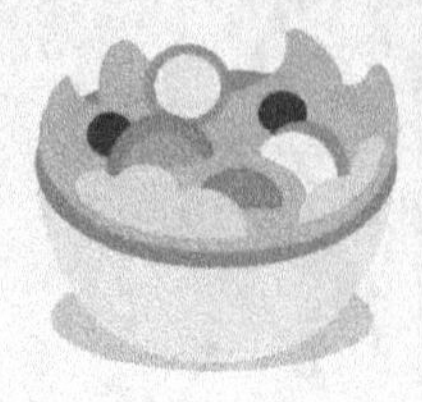

NAME: _________________________   DATE: _________________

FASTING DETAILS

FASTING START TIME: _____________________

FASTING END TIME: _____________________

TOTAL HOURS FASTED: _____________________

HOW DID YOU FEEL DURING YOUR FASTING PERIOD?
(ENERGY, MOOD, ANY CHALLENGES, ETC.)

HYDRATION TRACKER

TOTAL WATER INTAKE (CUPS): _____________________

ADDITIONAL BEVERAGES (TEA, HERBAL INFUSIONS, ETC.

PHYSICAL ACTIVITY

TYPE OF EXERCISE: _____________________________

DURATION: _____________________________

HOW DID IT FEEL?

MEALS & SNACKS LOG

TIME: _____________________

FOODS CONSUMED:

PORTION SIZE/COMMENTS

TIME: _____________________

FOODS CONSUMED:

PORTION SIZE/COMMENTS

Nutrition & Fasting Journal

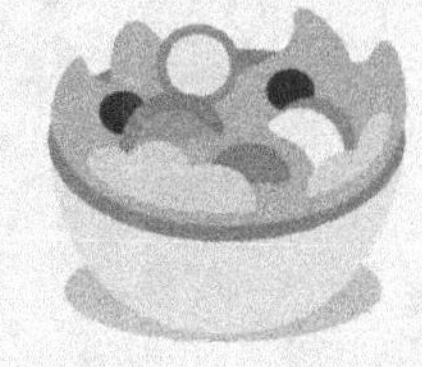

NAME: ________________   DATE: ____________

FASTING DETAILS
FASTING START TIME: ___________________
FASTING END TIME: ___________________
TOTAL HOURS FASTED: ___________________
HOW DID YOU FEEL DURING YOUR FASTING PERIOD?
(ENERGY, MOOD, ANY CHALLENGES, ETC.)

HYDRATION TRACKER
TOTAL WATER INTAKE (CUPS): ____________________
ADDITIONAL BEVERAGES (TEA, HERBAL INFUSIONS, ETC.)

PHYSICAL ACTIVITY
TYPE OF EXERCISE: ________________________________
DURATION: _____________________________
HOW DID IT FEEL?

MEALS & SNACKS LOG

TIME: ___________________
FOODS CONSUMED:
PORTION SIZE/COMMENTS

TIME: ___________________
FOODS CONSUMED:
PORTION SIZE/COMMENTS

Nutrition & Fasting Journal

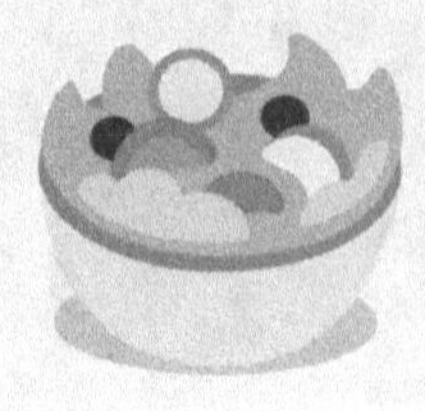

NAME: _________________________   DATE: _________________

FASTING DETAILS

FASTING START TIME: _____________________

FASTING END TIME: _____________________

TOTAL HOURS FASTED: _____________________

HOW DID YOU FEEL DURING YOUR FASTING PERIOD?
(ENERGY, MOOD, ANY CHALLENGES, ETC.)

HYDRATION TRACKER

TOTAL WATER INTAKE (CUPS): _____________________

ADDITIONAL BEVERAGES (TEA, HERBAL INFUSIONS, ETC.

PHYSICAL ACTIVITY

TYPE OF EXERCISE: _______________________________

DURATION: _______________________________

HOW DID IT FEEL?

MEALS & SNACKS LOG

TIME: ___________________

FOODS CONSUMED:
PORTION SIZE/COMMENTS

TIME: ___________________

FOODS CONSUMED:
PORTION SIZE/COMMENTS

Nutrition
& Fasting Journal

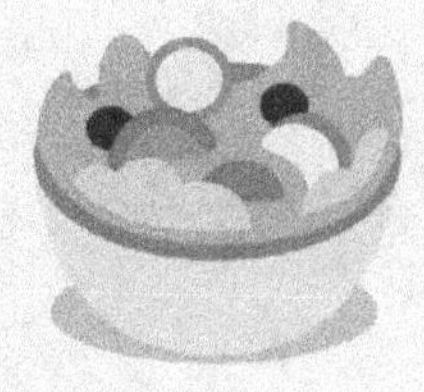

NAME: _________________   DATE: _______________

FASTING DETAILS
FASTING START TIME: _____________________
FASTING END TIME: _____________________
TOTAL HOURS FASTED: _____________________
HOW DID YOU FEEL DURING YOUR FASTING PERIOD?
(ENERGY, MOOD, ANY CHALLENGES, ETC.)

HYDRATION TRACKER
TOTAL WATER INTAKE (CUPS): _____________________
ADDITIONAL BEVERAGES (TEA, HERBAL INFUSIONS, ETC.)

PHYSICAL ACTIVITY
TYPE OF EXERCISE: _________________________________
DURATION: _________________________________
HOW DID IT FEEL?

MEALS & SNACKS LOG

TIME: _____________________
FOODS CONSUMED:
PORTION SIZE/COMMENTS

TIME: _________________
FOODS CONSUMED:
PORTION SIZE/COMMENTS

Conclusion

Celebrating Your Health Journey: A Symphony of Achievements

Think about all the milestones you've reached—big or small—and how each one adds a beautiful note to your unique health journey. Every nourishing meal, every workout, every moment of mindfulness has played a part in creating the vibrant, resilient life you enjoy today. Celebrate the determination that helped you overcome challenges and the perseverance that continues to drive your progress.

Reflecting on Progress: A Journey of Self-Discovery
Take a moment to look back on your path. Your progress isn't only visible in physical changes; it's also found in the deeper lessons learned along the way.

- **Discover the insights** about your body's needs and preferences.
- **Recognize the positive habits** you've built and the wisdom gained from setbacks.
- **Embrace the evolving relationship** you've

developed with your health and well-being.

Reflection is a strong tool that allows you to appreciate how far you've come while also preparing you to make thoughtful decisions in what is to come.

Embracing a Healthier Future: A Canvas of Possibilities

As you celebrate your achievements, look ahead with excitement. Picture your future as a blank canvas where every choice is a brushstroke, creating a masterpiece of well-being. **Refine your practices** by exploring new ways to nourish your body and mind.

128

Integrate fresh elements into
your routine to keep your journey
dynamic and fulfilling.
**Imagine a future filled with
vitality and joy**, where every step
you take builds on the foundation
of your progress.
This isn't the end—it's an
invitation to continue weaving
more threads into the tapestry of
your health.

As we conclude this journey
through intermittent fasting and
holistic well-being, especially
tailored for women over fifty, let's
embrace the idea of timeless
wellness.
Reflect on your journey—the

insights, habits, and wisdom you've gathered along the way. **See your health as a continuous process,** one that grows and evolves with you through the years. **Adopt practices that stand the test of time,** ensuring your well-being isn't just a momentary trend, but a lifelong commitment. Timeless wellness is about celebrating every stage of life, recognizing that health is an ongoing adventure that adapts to your changing needs.

www.ingramcontent.com/pod-product-compliance
Lightning Source LLC
Chambersburg PA
CBHW070849260726
48661CB00004B/1312